KETOGENIC DIET - Natural Treatment for Epilepsy and Other Disorders

The ultimate beginner's guide and cookbook

Table of Contents

Overview and History of Epilepsy

Ketogenic Diet and Epilepsy

Breakfast Ideas

Lunch Ideas

Dinner Ideas

Snack Ideas

Overview and History of Epilepsy

Epilepsy is usually defined as a neurological condition as well as a group of neurological disorders. It has been observed to have long term effects in the life of the affected individual. The episodes of seizures characterize this condition and they are one of its main symptoms.

The episodic occurrence of seizures is also the reason why some refer to this condition as a seizure disorder. Of course, there are other symptoms that help identify it but the seizures are the primary one. There are also psychosocial symptoms as well as postictal signs.

Note that the seizures that characterize this condition are actually symptoms of abnormal brain function. They usually last at different intervals. There are seizures that are only short and some are so brief that they tend to be unnoticeable. Other seizures can last longer, often with visible and vigorous shaking of the body.

In case of epileptic seizures, the actual cause of the abnormal brain function is categorized by experts as unidentifiable with the exception among the elderly and young children. That also brings in the discussion of demographics. Most of the time, it is likely that people know at least one individual (i.e. a family member, friend, or acquaintance) who has epilepsy.

It is estimated that 1% of people around the world have epilepsy. That accounts for around 65 million individuals. It should be noted that almost 80 percent of the cases of epilepsy are found in developing countries.

It should also be noted that the condition is observed to be more common as men and women grow older. If you check the statistics among developing countries, the occurrence of new epilepsy cases is more frequent among newborn children. Statistics also show that it is also just as common in people who are of retiring age.

The statistics for developing countries vary significantly. Note that new cases in such countries are actually more pronounced among older children as well as young adults. Hopefully, these numbers will one day help experts in the medical field.

There are differences with regard to the frequency of causes underlying this condition. It is estimated that around five percent to 10 percent of the entire worldwide population will experience an unprovoked seizure when they reach the age of 80. Estimates also show that the chances of having another seizure within this age group are between 40 percent and 50 percent.

It should be made clear that epilepsy itself is not a single disease. Instead it should be seen as more of a symptom. It is basically the result of a number of various diseases or disorders. Experts in the medical field are careful to distinguish epilepsy with other disorders or medical conditions that may have similar signs or symptoms.

In the case of actual epilepsy, the seizures are said to occur rather spontaneously. The seizure is said to occur without any sort of immediate cause, an example of which is an acute illness or some other probable health condition that can trigger seizures (e.g. an extreme drop in blood sugar levels etc.).

Some experts say that one of the possible underlying causes of epilepsy could very well be genetic. There are also others who believe that it is due to structural or metabolic problems. However, the rationale behind such conclusions is not 100% reliable.

That is also the reason why around 60% of epilepsy cases have unknown causes. Nevertheless, it has been observed that developmental conditions as well as genetic and congenital ones are usually observed in younger people. This observation is drawn along with the statistical figures mentioned earlier.

Congenital and genetic causes are usually ruled out as causes among older men and women. Doctors usually point to brain tumors and strokes as the more likely cause of this disorder among people in retiring ages. This distinction is usually clarified at the onset.

Other than specific symptoms and signs, there are factors that may contribute to the occurrence and development of seizures in a patient. Sometimes, they can very well occur as a consequence or result another health problem. These contributing factors can help doctors identify whether a patient's condition is actually epilepsy or not.

If seizures occur right after a patient experiences a certain or a specified cause, then it is usually referred to as an acute symptomatic seizure. Examples of said causes include a head injury, drug or alcohol misuse, stroke, brain cancer, an underlying metabolic problem, or the ingestion of other intoxicating substances. If this is the case, doctors usually rule out epilepsy and identify the condition as another kind of seizure related disorder. However, symptomatic seizures can also lead to other later seizures and that is when doctors will identify the case as a type of secondary epilepsy.

Ketogenic Diet and Epilepsy

There are several treatment options available for people with epilepsy. One of them is brain surgery, which is one of the more frightening prospects that the general public faces. Medical experts say that back in the day, a surgeon would wait for years, even decades, before recommending surgery for epilepsy patients. However, surgery procedures have become a lot better, safer, and more effective.

If surgery is still not an option for patients, then another treatment option that is less critical is a ketogenic diet. Medical experts have observed and have achieved success at treating this condition using this said diet. It's interesting that medical experts admit that it does work even though they do not know exactly how it works or why it works.

Much of the credence for ketogenic diets is due to its use as a successful treatment of children who suffer from severe epilepsy and are no longer responding to antiepileptic medication. In fact, medical experts have confirmed that this diet is a really effective treatment for any form of seizure that has been most probably caused by Lennox-Gastaut syndrome. Many parents of children with epilepsy opt for this treatment when all other treatments to control or manage a child's seizures have otherwise failed.

Overview of a Ketogenic Diet

The human body basically produces a substance known as ketones when it metabolizes body fat instead of carbohydrates. Everyone knows that the primary fuel of the human body is carbs. However, it is definitely possible, and it has been done by many populations of the world, where the body is taught to burn more fat instead of carbs.

That is basically the idea behind any ketogenic diet. This kind of diet forces the body to burn more body fat as the primary source of energy. Diets like this basically reduce or limit the amount of carbohydrates consumed by the patient and significantly increase the amount of fat being consumed.

That may sound strange to some people but it should be noted that there are people in the world who naturally thrive on a ketogenic diet. Eskimos have to live in climates where there aren't a lot of carbohydrate sources around. Their diets include a lot of fat and they basically live on ketogenic diets. This is evidence that living on such a diet is indeed possible.

But it is one thing to be naturally on a ketogenic diet and totally another to just induce one. The fact of the matter is that doctors usually recommend epilepsy patients to be admitted into a hospital before actually beginning the transition to a ketogenic diet. This is so that they can better monitor and care for a patient, especially if there is a serious underlying medical condition.

Once admitted, patients are made to fast one day and the night before actually beginning a ketogenic diet. Note that the approach is not like a crash diet where drastic dietary changes are made. In fact, the usual approach is to make gradual changes over time.

However, even though small changes are made to a person's diet, the person's body will see it as a dramatic change. This is one of the reasons why doctors prefer to have patients admitted first. During the first few days of a ketogenic diet, a patient may feel weak or at least feel a significant reduction in energy.

Doctors will primarily insist on having child patients admitted either to a hospital or an epileptic treatment center before commencing a ketogenic dietary change. The child will usually be under close observation. Often, a doctor or a dietician will supervise the provision of the said diet.

It should be noted at this point that ketogenic diets have been observed to be more successful in children than adults. But that doesn't mean an adult suffering from an epileptic condition will not get better by undergoing a ketogenic diet. It's just that the chances of success seem to be reduced as the patient gets older.

Doctors are baffled by this and there is still no solid explanation why this is so. It has been observed that four out of ten children who have undergone a ketogenic diet have a reduced number of seizure episodes, which is around 50 percent; some have even reduced the number of seizures to less than 50 percent.

A child on such a diet will only experience a quarter of the number of seizures of a child patient who has not gone through a ketogenic diet. These high success rates have been viewed as a sure sign of hope for parents and loved ones of patients around the world. This is also why many have opted for this treatment since it also helps the child or any other patient avoid the possible side effects of antiepileptic medication.

Nevertheless, it should be made clear that even something that seems simple as a ketogenic diet will also have its share of side effects. The people who try these diets sometimes report certain side effects, especially when they are just new to them. Nevertheless, the said side effects aren't always serious.

Some of the usual side effects or complaints that patients report include constipation, vomiting, dehydration, and a general feeling of weakness. Of course, there are more serious side effects that have been reported by patients and doctors as well. These include kidney stones, slower growth rates (usually observed among small children), increased cholesterol levels, and certain behavioral changes.

Other than the huge change in the type of food that patients eat, they are also given vitamin and mineral supplements. Since the usually available food sources have been reduced in this said diet, it eventually creates a deficiency in both the amount of vitamins and minerals that a person consumes. This is considered by some as another downside of ketogenic diets in general.

It should be noted at this point that there isn't a 100 percent support from the medical world about the use of ketogenic diets as a treatment for epilepsy. There are medical experts who are either critical of this treatment option or skeptical of its effectiveness. Most would recommend that a patient who undertakes a ketogenic diet should remain under the supervision of a doctor.

Remember that the health risks mentioned here are real, that includes the side effects that do not sound that serious. Health risks are still risks to any patient's health, especially if you're dealing with children. Such things should always be seriously considered in any situation involving a treatment for a serious condition.

Note that a patient must follow the recommendations of competent medical care providers in order to make ketogenic diets truly effective. That means the amount of food intake will be strict and precise. This makes these diets hard to follow at times.

Meal preparation for a ketogenic diet will usually take more time compared to meals that people cook up in the microwave. It should also be made clear that these diets aren't 100% fool proof. There is still a chance that it may not work for a patient even if a child is the subject of treatment and no matter how closely the recommendations are followed.

Admittedly, all medical experts agree that a ketogenic diet by itself is not a healthy diet to live on (thus the need for vitamin and mineral supplements). As always, with any epileptic treatment, proper care and information should be at the core before one decides to opt for a ketogenic diet.

Beginners' Ketogenic Diet Recipes

Breakfast Ideas

Lox and Avocado Crêpes

Prep Time: 10 minutes

Dehydrating Time: 7 - 10 hours

Servings: 2

INGREDIENTS

4 - 6 oz smoked salmon

1 ripe avocado

1/2 lemon

1 sprig fresh dill

1 teaspoon sesame seeds (black or white)

Crêpes

1 young coconut (plus coconut water)

1/3 cup raw sunflower seeds

1/2 cup flax seeds

1/2 white ground pepper (or 1/4 teaspoon ground black pepper)

1/2 teaspoon Celtic sea salt

Water

INSTRUCTIONS

1. For *Crêpes*, add flax to food processor or high-speed blender. Process until finely ground, up to 5 minutes. Add sunflower seeds and process until finely ground, about 1 minute.

2. Remove flesh and water from young coconut. Add to processor with salt and pepper. Process until smooth batter forms, about 1 - 2 minutes. Add enough water to reach desired consistency.

3. Place parchment paper or dehydrator sheets on dehydrator trays.

4. Spread batter on prepared sheets. Place trays in dehydrator and set to 115 degrees F for 6 - 8 hours.

5. Remove trays from dehydrator. Remove *Crepes* from parchment or dehydrator liners, flip, and place directly on dehydrator tray. Place trays back in dehydrator and continue dehydrating 1 - 2 hours, until surface is dry but *Crêpe* is still pliable.

6. Remove from dehydrator and cut into desired shape and size. Set aside.

7. Finely chop fresh dill. Cut avocado in half and remove pit. Slice flesh in peel.

8. Lay *Crêpes* flat and top with line of smoked salmon down center. Scoop portion of sliced avocado over smoked salmon. Sprinkle on chopped dill. Roll up *Crêpes* and transfer to serving dish.

9. Top *Crêpes* with squeeze of lemon juice and sprinkle on sesame seeds. Serve immediately.

Turkey Jerky Bacon

Prep Time: 10 minutes*

Dehydrating Time: 4 - 8 hours

Servings: 4

INGREDIENTS

4 oz organic turkey (dark meat)

2 tablespoons coconut aminos (or liquid aminos)

2 tablespoons tamari (or liquid aminos or coconut aminos)

1 tablespoon lemon juice (or raw apple cider vinegar)

1 tablespoons Celtic sea salt

1/2 teaspoon garlic powder

1/2 teaspoon onion powder

1/2 teaspoon smoked paprika

Pinch cayenne pepper

INSTRUCTIONS

1. Prepare two sheet parchment. Lay one on cutting board.
2. Cut turkey into 1/4 inch strips and lay in single layer on parchment. Pound with tenderizing side of kitchen mallet. Cover turkey with second parchment sheet, then pound with flat side of tenderizing mallet to 1/8 inch thickness.
3. *Place turkey strips in medium mixing bowl or shallow dish. Add coconut aminos, tamari, lemon juice, salt and spices. Mix well to coat. Cover and place in refrigerator for 8 hours, or overnight.

4. Remove turkey from refrigerator and lay in single layer on dehydrator trays. Place trays in dehydrator and set to 120 degrees F for 4 - 8 hours.

5. After 4 hours dehydrating time, remove trays from dehydrator and test turkey by bending. If it cracks, remove and serve immediately. Or store in airtight container.

6. If still flexible, place back in dehydrator and continue dehydrating up to 4 hours, or until desired texture is achieved.

Stone-wrought Coop

Prep time: 5 minutes

Cook time: 3-6 minutes

INGREDIENTS

2 cage-free eggs

1 small onion

1 clove garlic

½ red bell pepper

1 tbsp extra virgin olive oil

¼ tsp smoked paprika

¼ tsp ground black pepper

INSTRUCTIONS

1. Finely chop onion, garlic and red bell pepper.
2. Pour extra virgin olive oil into a pan over medium heat.
3. Crack eggs and pour into a small bowl. Combine with onion, garlic and red bell pepper and whisk until mixed together.
4. Pour contents of bowl into pan and add smoked paprika and ground black pepper. Scramble until desired doneness. Serve.

Ancient Egg Muffins

Prep time: 5 minutes

Cook time: 15-20 minutes

INGREDIENTS

1 tbsp olive oil

1 tbsp coconut oil

6 cage-free eggs

1 onion

½ yellow bell pepper

½ red bell pepper

¼ tsp ground black pepper

¼ tsp Celtic sea salt

INSTRUCTIONS

1. Preheat oven to 350. Whisk all 6 eggs in a bowl. Chop the onion and bell pepper into small pieces.
2. In a pan, combine olive oil with onion over medium-high heat for 2 minutes. Add peppers and cook another 2 minutes.
3. Remove onion/peppers from heat and let cool a few minutes. Combine them with the eggs. Add the Celtic sea salt and ground black pepper and mix.
4. Coat a muffin pan with the coconut oil. Fill each muffin cup with the egg/pepper/onion mix. Do not fill a muffin cup more than ¾ full.

5. Place the pan in the oven and bake 10-15 minutes, removing the pan from the oven when the tops of the muffins get fluffy and golden brown.

6. Remove the muffins from the pan and serve.

Sizzled Chicken Wraps

Prep time: 5 minutes

Cook time: 3 minutes

INGREDIENTS

4 slices of chicken deli meat

1 tbsp olive oil

1 small onion

1 red bell pepper

1 avocado

¼ tsp garlic powder

INSTRUCTIONS

1. Remove the nut from the avocado and mash it into a paste. Chop the pepper and onion into small pieces.
2. Combine the garlic powder, pepper and onion in the bowl with the avocado and mix well.
3. Add the olive oil in a pan over low heat and heat the chicken mildly, turning frequently, for 3 minutes.
4. Remove the chicken from heat and place ¼ of the avocado/pepper/onion mixture onto each piece.
5. Wrap the chicken up into tubes and serve.

Green Monster Kale and Poached Eggs

Prep time: 10 minutes

Cook time: 12 minutes

INGREDIENTS

1 handful kale

2 cage-free eggs

1 small onion

1 clove garlic

1 tbsp extra virgin olive oil

¼ tsp ground black pepper

1 tsp low-sodium horseradish (optional)

INSTRUCTIONS

1. Chop the onion and mince the garlic. De-stem and wash the kale. Leaving a bit of water on the kale is ideal.

2. In a saucepan, add 1 tbsp extra virgin olive oil over medium heat. Add onion and cook until it begins to lose its opaqueness, about 5 minutes.

3. Add kale to saucepan and cover until kale is soft and green, about 5 minutes. Add garlic and stir, then cook another 2 minutes and remove from heat.

4. Fill a saucepan half full of water. Bring the water to a boil, then reduce heat below a boil and hold it there.

5. One by one, crack the eggs into a small cup or bowl and, with the lip of the cup or bowl close to the water's surface, dump the egg

into the water. If necessary, nudge the eggwhites closer to the yolks to keep them together.

6. Once all the eggs are in the water, remove the pan from heat and cover it. Let sit for 4 minutes until all eggs are cooked, then remove eggs from pan.

7. Place the greens on a plate and the two eggs on top of the greens. Top with horseradish if desired. Serve.

Lunch Ideas

Mexican Tomato Soup

Prep Time: 35 minutes

Servings: 2

INGREDIENTS

Shrimp

10 - 12 large shrimp

1 - 1 1/2 cups lemon juice (about 8 lemons)

1/2 jalapeño pepper

Gazpacho

2 cups tomato juice (about 4 large tomatoes)

2 plum tomatoes

1/2 red bell pepper

1/2 red onion

1/2 cucumber

Small bunch fresh cilantro

2 garlic cloves

2 tablespoons raw apple cider vinegar(optional)

2 tablespoons raw oil (coconut, walnut, almond, sesame, etc.) (optional)

1 teaspoon ground black pepper

1 teaspoon Celtic sea salt

INSTRUCTIONS

1. For *Shrimp*, Peel, devein and remove tails from shrimp. Mince jalapeño and juice lemons. Add to small bowl and mix. Shrimp should be completely covered in lemon juice. Place in refrigerator for 30 minutes, or until shrimp are opaque.

2. For Gazpacho, juice large tomatoes in juicer. Or add to food processor or high-speed blender and process, then strain into medium mixing bowl.

3. Peel cucumber and seed. Seed plum tomatoes. Seed, stem and vein bell peppers. Peel onion and garlic. Dice veggies and onion, and mince garlic. Add to tomato juice.

4. Add salt, pepper, vinegar and oil (optional). Mix well, then place in refrigerator.

5. Chop cilantro and set aside.

6. Remove shrimp from refrigerator and drain lemon juice and jalapeños. Rinse if desired.

7. Mix shrimp into tomato mixture. Pour into serving bowls and top with chopped cilantro. Serve chilled.

Texas Chili

Prep Time: 10 minutes*

Servings: 2

INGREDIENTS

5 - 6 plum tomatoes

1/2 teaspoon dried cumin

1/4 teaspoon chili powder

1/4 teaspoon onion powder

1/4 teaspoon garlic powder

1 teaspoon fresh oregano leaves (or 1/4 teaspoon dried oregano)

1/2 teaspoon ground black pepper

1/4 teaspoon cayenne pepper or red pepper flakes (optional)

1 teaspoon Celtic sea salt

1 teaspoon chia seed (or flax seed)

1/2 cup raw cashews

Water

INSTRUCTIONS

1. *Soak raw cashews in enough water to cover overnight in refrigerator. Drain and rinse. Set aside.

2. Grind chia or flax in food processor or high-speed blender. Set aside.

3. Juice tomatoes. Or add to food processor or high-speed blender and process. Add enough water to reach desired consistency, if necessary. Then strain.

4. Add tomato juice, ground chia or flax, 1/2 of soaked cashews, salt, pepper and spices to blender. Process until smooth, about 1 - 2 minutes.
5. Stir in remaining soaked cashews.
6. Pour into serving bowls and serve immediately.

Creamy "Cheese" and Broccoli Soup

Prep Time: 10 minutes*

Servings: 2

INGREDIENTS

1 1/2 - 2 cups broccoli florets

1 red bell pepper

1 garlic clove

1/4 cup raw oil (coconut, walnut, almond, sesame, etc.)

1 cup nutritional yeast

1 tablespoon coconut aminos (or tamari)

1 tablespoon onion powder

1/2 teaspoon Celtic sea salt

1/4 teaspoon ground white pepper (or ground black pepper)

2 cups raw cashews

Water

INSTRUCTIONS

1. * Soak raw cashews in enough water to cover at least 2 hours, or overnight in refrigerator. Drain and rinse. Set aside.
2. Chop broccoli florets into pieces and set aside.
3. Seed and vein bell pepper. Peel garlic. Add to food processor or high-speed blender with soaked cashews, nutritional yeast, coconut aminos, salt, pepper and enough water to process until smooth, about 2 - 3 minutes.
4. Pour into serving bowl and top with broccoli. Serve immediately.

Caesar Salad

Prep Time: 10 minutes

Servings: 1

INGREDIENTS

2 cups chopped romaine lettuce

Almond Parmesan

1/4 cup raw almonds

1 teaspoon raw apple cider vinegar

1 teaspoon nutritional yeast (optional)

1/4 teaspoon garlic powder

1/4 teaspoon onion powder

1/4 teaspoon dried oregano

1/4 teaspoon Celtic sea salt

Raw Caesar Dressing

2 tablespoons raw cashews (or raw sunflower seeds)

2 tablespoons raw sunflower seeds

1 tablespoon raw pine nuts (or raw sesame seeds or raw tahini)

2 tablespoons lemon juice

1 garlic clove

3/4 teaspoon coconut aminos (or nutritional yeast)

1/2 teaspoon dried dill (optional)

Cracked or ground black pepper, to taste

Water

INSTRUCTIONS

1. Rinse, dry and plate romaine lettuce.

2. For *Almond Parmesan*, add almonds, vinegar, salt, spices and nutritional yeast (optional) to food processor or high-speed blender. Process until almonds are coarsely ground and resemble ground parmesan cheese. Set aside.

3. For *Raw Caesar Dressing*, peel garlic and add to food processor or high-speed blender with lemon juice. Process until smooth. Then add remaining ingredients and process until smooth, about 1 - 2 minutes. Add enough water to reach desired consistency.

4. Drizzle *Raw Caesar Dressing* over salad and sprinkle with *Almond Parmesan*. Serve immediately.

Smoked Salmon Avocado Salad

Prep Time: 10 minutes

Servings: 1

INGREDIENTS

Salad

2 cups soft lettuce leaves (looseleaf or butterhead varieties)

1/2 cup watercress or dandelion leaves (optional)

2 oz smoked salmon

1/2 avocado

1 sprig fresh dill

1 tablespoon caviar (optional)

Avocado Cream Dressing

1/2 avocado

1 sprig fresh dill

1 tablespoon lemon juice

1/2 teaspoon ground black pepper

1/2 teaspoon Celtic sea salt

1/2 coconut

Water

INSTRUCTIONS

1. For *Salad*, rinse, dry and plate lettuce and watercress or dandelion leaves (optional). Cut avocado in half and remover pit. Dice or slice avocado flesh in peel, then scoop onto greens. Lay smoked salmon over greens.

2. For *Avocado Cream Dressing*, remove coconut flesh from peel and add to food processor or high-speed blender with enough water to reach desired consistency. Process until smooth and creamy, about 1 - 2 minutes. Strain mixture through nut milk bag and place back into blender.

3. Scoop remaining avocado flesh into blender. Add lemon juice, 1 sprig dill, salt and pepper and process until well combined and smooth, about 1 minute.

4. Drizzle *Avocado Cream Dressing* over salad. Mince remaining dill and sprinkle over salad. Dollop caviar over salad (optional).

5. Serve immediately.

Pesto Tomato Caprese

Prep Time: 5 minutes

Servings: 2

INGREDIENTS

1 large yellow tomato

1 large red tomato

Small bunch fresh basil

Celtic sea salt, to taste

Crack or ground black pepper, to taste

Basil Pesto

2 cups basil leaves (packed)

1/4 cup raw pine nuts

1/2 - 1/3 cup raw oil (coconut, walnut, almond, sesame, etc.)

2 garlic cloves

1/2 lemon (or 1 tablespoon raw apple cider vinegar)

1/4 teaspoon Celtic sea salt

INSTRUCTIONS

1. For *Basil Pesto*, peel garlic and add to food processor or high-speed blender with squeeze of 1/2 lemon. Process until finely chopped. Add pine nuts, basil, oil and salt and process until finely ground, about 1 minute.
2. Slice tomatoes and plate in alternating colors. Sprinkle with salt and pepper. Chiffon basil leaves.

3. Spread *Basil Pesto* over tomato slices and top with fresh basil. Serve immediately.

Cilantro Taco Salad

Prep Time: 10 minutes

Servings: 1

INGREDIENTS

Salad

2 cups lettuce (chopped)

1/2 cup cilantro (chopped)

1 plum tomato

1/2 small onion

1 garlic clove

1 avocado

1/2 lime

1/2 jalapeño

Paprika, to taste

Ground black pepper, to taste

Celtic sea salt, to taste

Raw Taco Meat

1/4 cup walnuts

2 - 3 sundried tomatoes

1/4 teaspoon cumin

1/8 teaspoon garlic powder

1/8 teaspoon smoked paprika

1/8 teaspoon ground white pepper (or ground black pepper)

1/8 teaspoon teaspoon Celtic sea salt

INSTRUCTIONS

1. For *Salad*, rinse, dry and plate lettuce and cilantro. Reserve pinch of cilantro in small mixing bowl.

2. Peel onion and dice. Reserve 1/2 of onion in separate mixing bowl and add remaining onion to reserved cilantro. Remove seeds from jalapeño ad mince. Dice tomato. Add to onion and cilantro with squeeze of lime. Sprinkle on pinch of salt and pepper, and mix to combine. Set aside.

3. Cut avocado in half and remove pit. Scoop flesh into bowl with reserved onion. Peel garlic and mince, and add to avocado with squeeze of lime. Sprinkle on salt, pepper and paprika to taste. Mash slightly and mix with fork until well combine but still chunky. Set aside.

4. For *Raw Taco Meat*, add walnuts, sundried tomatoes, salt, pepper and spices to food processor or high-speed blender. Pulse until coarsely ground.

5. Top *Salad* with *Raw Taco Meat*, avocado and tomato mix. Serve immediately.

Asian Shrimp Lettuce Wraps

Prep Time: 35 minutes

Servings: 2

INGREDIENTS

4 large lettuce leaves (thin, flexible ribs)

1 cup cabbage (shredded)

1 small carrot

1/2 green onion

1/2 inch piece fresh ginger

1 small garlic clove

1/2 teaspoon raw sesame seeds

1/2 teaspoon coconut aminos (or tamari or raw apple cider vinegar)

1 teaspoon raw oil (sesame, coconut, walnut, almond, etc.)

Shrimp

10 - 12 medium shrimp

3/4 cup lemon juice (about 5 lemons)

1 teaspoon red pepper flakes

1/2 green onion (scallion)

Almond Sauce

2 tablespoons raw oil (sesame, coconut, walnut, almond, etc.)

1/4 cup raw almond butter (or 1/2 cup raw almonds)

1 tablespoon lemon juice (or coconut aminos or tamari)

1/2 small mild chili pepper

Water

INSTRUCTIONS

1. For *Shrimp*, slice green onion and reserve half in small mixing bowl. Peel, devein and remove tails from shrimp. Add to separate bowl with lemon juice, remaining green onion and red pepper. Mix to combine. Shrimp should be completely covered in lemon juice. Place in refrigerator for 30 minutes, or until shrimp are opaque.

2. Peel ginger and garlic, and finely grate or mince. Add to green onion with coconut aminos and oil. Mix to combine. Set aside.

3. For *Almond Sauce*, add oil, almond butter or almonds, lemon juice and chili pepper to food processor or high-speed blender. Process until smooth and creamy, about 1 - 2 minutes. Add enough water to reach desired consistency. Transfer to serving dish.

4. Shred cabbage and carrot and add to ginger mixture. Toss to coat.

5. Rinse, dry and plate lettuce leaves. Drain shrimp and layer onto lettuce. Top with cabbage mixture and sprinkle on sesame seeds. Roll up lettuce wraps and serve with *Almond Sauce*.

Chicken Fries with Garlic Aioli

Prep Time: 10 minutes

Cook Time: 15 minutes

Servings: 2

INGREDIENTS

8 oz boneless, skinless chicken breast

1 egg

1/2 cup almond meal

1 teaspoon flax meal (or ground chia seed)

1 teaspoon ground black pepper

1/2 teaspoon paprika

1/2 teaspoon onion powder

1/2 teaspoon garlic powder

1/2 teaspoon chili powder

1/2 teaspoon sea salt

Garlic Aioli

1/2 - 3/4 cup coconut oil

1 egg yolk

2 garlic cloves

1/2 small lemon

1/4 teaspoon ground white pepper (or black pepper)

1/4 teaspoon sea salt

3 tablespoons flavorful oil (black truffle, walnut, almond, sesame, etc.) (optional)

INSTRUCTIONS

1. Heat large pan over medium-high heat and coat with coconut oil.

2. For *Garlic Aioli*, peel garlic and add to food processor or blender with egg yolk, juice of 1/2 lemon, salt and pepper. Process until smooth, scraping down sides of vessel.

3. While processor or blender is running, very slowly drizzle in enough coconut oil to create thick mayo-like mixture. Drizzle in flavorful oil as well will processor runs (optional). If mixture is runny, drizzle in more coconut oil while processor runs until thickened. Pour into serving dish and refrigerate.

4. Slice chicken into half width-wise, creating twice the fillets. Try to slice at thickest portion to keep all fillets equal thickness.

5. Slice chicken fillets into long, 1/2 inch wide strips. Place strips between two paper towels and press to absorb excess moisture.

6. In a shallow dish, blend almond meal, flax or chia meal, spices and salt.

7. Beat egg in small mixing bowl. Toss chicken strips in beaten egg to lightly coat, then dredge in seasoned almond meal.

8. Carefully place coated chicken strips into hot oil and fry about 2 - 3 minutes, until golden brown and cooked through. Turn with tongs half way through cooking.

9. Drain cooked chicken on paper towel, then transfer to serving dish.

10. Serve hot with *Garlic Aioli*.

Quick Chili

Prep Time: 5 minutes

Cook Time: 20 minutes

Servings: 4

INGREDIENTS

1 lb lean grass-fed ground beef (or elk, bison, turkey or chicken)

15 oz (1 can) organic tomato sauce

6 oz (1 can) organic tomato paste

1 small onion

1 bell pepper

2 cloves garlic

2 tablespoons chili powder

1 tablespoon ground cumin

1 tablespoon smoked paprika (or paprika)

1 teaspoon Mexican oregano (or dried oregano)

1 teaspoon ground black pepper

1 teaspoon sea salt

1/2 teaspoon cayenne pepper

1 tablespoon coconut oil

sea salt, to taste

INSTRUCTIONS

1. Heat medium pot over medium-high heat. Add 1 tablespoon coconut oil.

2. Peel onion and garlic. Stem and seed bell pepper. Chop and add to food processor or bullet blender. Pulse until finely minced.

3. Add to skillet and sauté for about 1 minute. Add ground beef and spices. Brown beef for about 5 minutes. Stir with whisk to break up meat well, or wooden spoon to keep beef chunkier.

4. Add whole cans of tomato sauce and paste. Stir to combine.

5. Bring to a simmer, then reduce heat to medium and cover loosely with lid to prevent splatter. Simmer about 10 minutes. Stir occasionally.

6. Use large serving spoon or ladle to serve hot.

Dinner Ideas

Zucchini Pasta with Sundried Tomato Sauce

Prep Time: 5 minutes

Servings: 2

INGREDIENTS

1 large zucchini

Zesty Tomato Sauce

2 medium tomatoes (or 3 plum tomatoes)

5 sundried tomatoes

2 tablespoons raw cashews (or 1 tablespoon raw cashew butter)

2 large garlic cloves

Small bunch fresh basil leaves

1 small fresh oregano sprig

Ground black pepper, to taste

Cayenne pepper, to taste

Celtic sea salt, to taste

INSTRUCTIONS

1. Carefully slice zucchini with spiralizer, vegetable peeler, or sharp knife. Sprinkle with pinch of salt, pepper and cayenne. Gently toss to coat and set aside.

2. For *Zesty Tomato Sauce*, remove basil and oregano leaves from stems. Peel garlic. Add to food processor or high-speed blender with tomatoes, sundried tomatoes, cashews or cashew butter, salt, pepper and cayenne. Process until smooth, about 1 - 2 minutes.

3. Transfer zucchini pasta to serving dishes. Top with *Zesty Tomato Sauce* and serve immediately.

Zucchini Pasta with Pesto

Prep Time: 10 minutes

Servings: 2

INGREDIENTS

1 small zucchini

1 bell pepper (or 1 carrot)

Pine Nut Pesto

2 1/2 cups fresh basil leaves

1/2 cup raw pine nuts

1 garlic clove

2 tablespoons raw oil (walnut, almond, coconut, sesame, etc.)

1/4 teaspoon ground white pepper (or ground black pepper)

1/4 teaspoon Celtic sea salt

INSTRUCTIONS

1. Carefully slice zucchini with spiralizer, vegetable peeler, or sharp knife. Carefully slice carrot with spiralizer, vegetable peeler, or grater, if using. Or remove stem, seeds and veins from bell pepper, then julienne (cut into long thin slices). Set aside.

2. For *Pine Nut Pesto*, peel garlic and add to food processor or high-speed blender with basil, 2 tablespoons pine nuts, oil, salt and pepper. Process until thick, smooth mixture forms, about 1 - 2 minutes.

3. Add *Pine Nut Pesto* to veggie pasta and toss to coat. Transfer to serving dish and top with remaining pine nuts. Serve immediately.

Zucchini Fettuccini Alfredo

Prep Time: 10 minutes

Servings: 2

INGREDIENTS

1 medium zucchini

1 carrot (or 1 small sweet potato)

Alfredo Sauce

1 cup raw cashews

1 teaspoon lemon juice (or raw apple cider vinegar)

2 garlic cloves

1/2 teaspoon dried thyme

1/2 teaspoon Celtic sea salt

Water

Walnut Parmesan

1/2 cup raw walnuts

3 tablespoons nutritional yeast

1/4 teaspoon ground white pepper (or ground black pepper)

1/2 teaspoon Celtic sea salt

INSTRUCTIONS

1. Carefully slice zucchini and carrot or sweet potato with spiralizer, vegetable peeler, or grater. Set aside.

2. For *Alfredo Sauce*, peel garlic and add to food processor or high-speed blender with cashews, lemon juice, thyme and salt. Process

until smooth mixture forms, up to 5 minutes. Add enough water to reach desired consistency. Set aside.

3. For *Walnut Parmesan*, add walnuts to clean food processor or high-speed blender and process until finely ground. Add nutritional yeast, salt and pepper. Process until coarsely ground and mixture resembling parmesan cheese forms.

4. Add *Alfredo Sauce* to veggie pasta and toss to coat. Transfer to serving dish and top with *Walnut Parmesan*. Serve immediately.

Cashew Crunch Kelp Noodle Salad

Prep Time: 10 minutes*

Servings: 2

INGREDIENTS

1 package (12 oz) kelp noodles

1/2 lemon

1/2 small red bell pepper

Cashew Sauce

1 cup raw cashews

1/2 small red bell pepper

1/2 lemon

1 tablespoon coconut aminos (or raw apple cider vinegar)

2 large basil leaves

1/2 teaspoon smoked paprika

1/2 teaspoon ground black pepper

1/2 teaspoon Celtic sea salt

1/4 teaspoon ground turmeric (optional)

1/4 teaspoon smoked chili powder (optional)

Water

INSTRUCTIONS

1. *Soak 3/4 cup cashews in enough water to cover at least 4 hours, or overnight in refrigerator. Drain and rinse.

2. Drain and rinse kelp noodles. Add to medium bowl with warm water and juice of 1/2 lemon. Set aside 5 minutes.

3. Cut bell pepper in half. Remove stem, seeds and veins and set half of pepper aside. Julienne (thinly slice) remaining bell pepper and add to medium mixing bowl.

5. For *Crunchy Cashew Sauce*, add soaked cashews, bell pepper, juice of 1/2 lemon, coconut aminos, basil, salt and spices to food processor or high-speed blender. Process until smooth, about 2 minutes. Add enough water to reach desired consistency. Set aside.

4. Drain kelp noodles and add to sliced bell pepper. Add *Cashew Sauce* and toss to coat. Transfer noodles to serving dishes.

5. Roughly chop remaining 1/4 cup cashews. Sprinkle noodles and serve immediately. Or refrigerate for 20 minutes and serve chilled.

Raw Walnuts Tacos

Prep Time: 35 minutes

Servings: 2

INGREDIENTS

4 large lettuce leaves (thin, flexible ribs)

1 plum tomato

1/4 red onion (or white or yellow onion)

Medium bunch cilantro

1 avocado

1/2 lime

Taco Meat

1 cup raw walnuts

1/2 cup sundried tomatoes

1/2 teaspoon ground cumin

1/4 teaspoon garlic powder

1/4 teaspoon smoked chili powder

1/4 teaspoon Celtic sea salt

Cayenne pepper, to taste

Cashew Sour Cream

1/2 cup raw cashews

1 lemon

1/8 teaspoon Celtic sea salt

3 tablespoons cup water

1/3 cup ice

INSTRUCTIONS

6. *Soak sundried tomatoes in enough water to cover at least 2 hours, or overnight in refrigerator. Drain.

7. For *Taco Meat*, add soaked tomatoes, walnuts, salt and spices to food processor or high-speed blender. Process until chunky mixture forms, about 1 minute. Set aside

8. For *Cashew Sour Cream*, add cashews, lemon juice, salt, water and ice to clean food processor or high-speed blender. Process until smooth, about 2 minutes.

9. Chop cilantro. Dice tomato. Thinly slice onion. Cut avocado in half, then remove pit and slice in peel.

10. Fill lettuce leaves with *Taco Meat*. Scoop avocado slices onto *Taco Meat*. Drizzle on *Cashew Sour Cream*. Top with diced onion and tomato, and sprinkle of chopped cilantro. Top with squeeze of lime.

11. Fold lettuce around filling and transfer to serving dish. Serve immediately.

Tilapia Lettuce Wraps

Prep Time: 35 minutes

Servings: 2

INGREDIENTS

1 lb boneless, skinless tilapia fillets (or other white fish)

1 1/4 cup lemon juice (about 8 lemons)

4 large lettuce leaves (thin, flexible ribs)

1 cup cabbage (shredded)

1 small carrot

1/2 green onion (scallion)

Cilantro Sauce

1/2 cup raw cashews

1 lemon

1/2 inch piece fresh ginger

1 small garlic clove

Medium bunch cilantro

1/4 teaspoon Celtic sea salt

3 tablespoons water

1/3 cup ice

INSTRUCTIONS

1. Juice lemons into medium mixing bowl. Cut tilapia into 1 inch strips. Add to lemon juice and toss to coat. Tilapia should be completely covered in lemon juice. Place in refrigerator for 30 minutes, or until tilapia is opaque.

2. Carefully slice carrot with spiralizer, vegetable peeler, or grater. Shred cabbage. Slice green onion. Set aside.

3. For *Cilantro Sauce*, remove cilantro leaves form stems. Peel ginger and garlic. Add to food processor or high-speed blender with cashews, lemon juice, salt, water and ice. Process until smooth, about 2 minutes.

4. Remove tilapia from refrigerator and drain. Gently rinse, if preferred. Fill lettuce leaves wit tilapia. Add shredded cabbage and carrot. Drizzle on *Cilantro Sauce*. Top with sliced green onions.

5. Fold lettuce around filling and transfer to serving dish. Serve immediately.

City Clam Chowder

Prep Time: 35 minutes

Servings: 2

INGREDIENTS

2 dozen live littleneck clams

1 - 1 1/2 cups lemon juice (about 8 lemons)

2 cups tomato juice (about 4 large tomatoes)

2 plum tomatoes

1 celery stalk

1 carrot

1 red bell pepper

1 green bell pepper

1/4 teaspoon cayenne pepper

1/2 teaspoon onion powder

1 teaspoon dried oregano

1 teaspoon dried basil

1 teaspoon ground black pepper

1 teaspoon Celtic sea salt

INSTRUCTIONS

5. Have fishmonger shuck clams. Or carefully shuck clams yourself. Reserve clam juice.

6. Juice lemons into medium mixing bowl. Add clams and toss to coat. Clams should be completely covered in lemon juice. Place in refrigerator for 30 minutes, or until clams are opaque.

7. Juice large tomatoes in juicer then add to food processor or high-speed blender. Or add to food processor or high-speed blender and process, then strain and return to processor.

8. Remove stems, seeds and veins from bell peppers. Cut red and green bell pepper in half. Cut carrot and celery stalks in half. Add half of each veggie to tomato juice with salt and spices. Process until smooth, about 2 minutes. Add to medium mixing bowl. Set aside.

9. Dice plum tomatoes, and remaining celery, carrot, and bell pepper. Add to tomato purée with reserved clam juice, salt and spices.

10. Remove clams from refrigerator and drain lemon juice. Gently rinse, if desired. Add to bowl and mix to combine.

11. Transfer to serving dish and serve immediately.

Creamy French Onion Soup

Prep Time: 15 minutes*

Dehydrating Time: 6 hours

Servings: 2

INGREDIENTS

3 cups raw almond milk (or 1 cup raw almonds + 4 cups water)

1/2 lemon

1/4 cup tamari (or coconut aminos or raw apple cider vinegar)

1 tablespoon coconut aminos (or tamari or raw apple cider vinegar)

2 tablespoons raw oil or butter (ghee, cacao butter, coconut butter, almond oil, walnut oil, coconut oil, etc.)

1/2 teaspoon dried thyme

1/2 teaspoon cracked black pepper (or ground black pepper)

Caramelized Onions

2 onions

1 tablespoon raw honey (or 2 dried pitted dates)

1 tablespoon tamari (or coconut aminos or raw apple cider vinegar)

1 tablespoon raw oil (almond, walnut, coconut, etc.)

1/4 teaspoon Celtic sea salt

INSTRUCTIONS

1. *Soak almonds in 1 cup water at least 6 hours, or overnight in refrigerator. Drain and pop off skins, if preferred.

2. For *Caramelized Onions*, add dates, tamari, oil and salt to food processor or high-speed blender and process until smooth. Add water to reach desired consistency, if necessary.

3. Or add honey, tamari, oil and salt to large mixing bowl and mix to combine. Peel onions and thinly slice. Add to bowl and toss to coat.

4. Prepare several dehydrator or parchment sheets and line dehydrator tray. Spread coated onion on prepared trays and place in dehydrator on 110 degrees F for 6 hours.

5. Add soaked almonds to high-speed blender with 3 cups water. Process until well blended and almost smooth, about 1-2 minutes.

6. Strain mixture through nut milk bag, cheesecloth or strainer back into processor. Reserve almond pulp and dehydrate for almond flour.

7. Add juice of 1/2 lemon, coconut aminos, tamari, oil, thyme and black pepper to almond milk. Add half of *Caramelized Onions* and process until smooth, about 1 minute.

8. Add half of remaining *Caramelized Onions* and pulse until onions are roughly chopped.

9. Transfer to serving dish and top with remaining *Caramelized Onions*. Serve immediately.

Salmon Tartar Stack

Prep Time: 10 minutes*

Servings: 2

INGREDIENTS

8 oz boneless, skinless salmon fillet (sushi grade)

2 limes

1 avocado

1 shallot

1 tablespoon raw oil (coconut, walnut, almond, sesame, etc.)

1 teaspoon mustard seeds (or ground mustard)

Medium sprig fresh dill

Celtic sea salt, to taste

Ground black pepper, to taste

2 teaspoons caviar (optional)

INSTRUCTIONS

1. Have fishmonger prepare salmon fillets. Or fillet salmon and remove pin bones and skin.

2. Dice salmon and transfer to serving dish. Top with squeeze of 1/2 lime and sprinkle of salt and pepper. Place in mold to form, if preferred.

3. Peel and thinly slice shallot, then add to small mixing bowl. Juice whole lime into food processor or high-speed blender. Add oil, mustard seeds and pinch of salt and pepper. Process to combine, then add to shallots.

4. Or add lime juice, oil, ground mustard, salt and pepper to shallots. Mix to combine and set aside.

5. Cut avocado in half and remove pit. Dice flesh in peel and scoop into separate mixing bowl. Finely chop dill and add to avocado with squeeze of remaining 1/2 lime, salt and pepper. Mix to combine.

6. Add avocado dill mixture to salmon. Then top with shallot mixture and caviar (optional). Serve immediately.

7. *Or refrigerate 2 hours and serve chilled.

Simple Steak Tartar

Prep Time: 10 minutes*

Servings: 2

INGREDIENTS

10 oz beef tenderloin

Small bunch fresh parsley

1/2 lemon

2 cage-free egg yolk (optional)

2 tablespoons raw oil (coconut, walnut, almond, sesame, etc.)

1 teaspoon ground mustard (or mustard seeds)

1 shallot

1/4 teaspoon chili flakes (optional)

Ground black pepper, to taste

Celtic sea salt, to taste

INSTRUCTIONS

1. Finely dice tenderloin and parsley. Add to bowl with squeeze of lemon and pinch of salt and pepper. Mix to combine.
2. Transfer to serving dish. Place in ring mold to form, if preferred. Set aside.
3. Peel shallot and mince. Add to small mixing bowl with egg yolks (optional), mustard, oil, salt and spices. Whisk to emulsify.
4. Top tenderloin with mixture and serve immediately. Or refrigerate 20 minutes and serve chilled.

Macadamia Crusted Ahi Tuna

Prep Time: 5 minutes

Cook Time: 1 minute

Servings: 1

INGREDIENTS

8 oz ahi tuna fillet

1/4 teaspoon coconut oil

1/4 teaspoon dried thyme

1/4 teaspoon dried tarragon (optional)

1/4 cup whole macadamia nuts (shelled)

1 small garlic clove teaspoon

1 small shallot teaspoon

1/2 teaspoon ground white pepper (or black pepper)

1/2 teaspoon sea salt

2 tablespoons coconut oil

INSTRUCTIONS

1. Heat medium pan over medium-high heat. Add 2 tablespoons coconut oil to pan.
2. Chop macadamia nuts well. Peel and finely mince garlic and shallot. Set aside.
3. Rub top and bottom of fillet with 1/4 teaspoon coconut oil, salt, pepper, thyme and tarragon (optional).
4. Press 1/2 chopped macadamia nuts into each side of fillet.
5. Add garlic and shallots to hot oiled pan and sauté for just a second. Do not burn.

6. Carefully place fish in pan and sear 15 - 30 seconds on each side, for rare to medium rare. Carefully flip half way through cooking.
7. Transfer fillet to serving dish and serve hot with mixed greens or favorite veggies.

Parchment Baked Salmon

Prep Time: 5 minutes

Cook Time: 20 minutes

Servings: 1

INGREDIENTS

8 oz salmon fillet (deboned, skin-on)

6 - 8 medium asparagus stalks

1/2 lemon

1 basil sprig

1 rosemary sprig

1 teaspoon coconut oil

Pinch black pepper

Pinch sea salt

Parchment paper

Kitchen twine

INSTRUCTIONS

1. Place large sheet pan on bottom rack of oven. Preheat oven to 400 degrees F. prepare parchment sheet.

2. Place salmon in middle of parchment sheet skin-side down and sprinkle with salt and pepper. Place asparagus stalks next to salmon. Cut lemon into thin slices and place over fish and asparagus. Rub herbs between palms, then lay basil and rosemary sprig over lemon slices. Drizzle 1 teaspoon coconut oil over salmon and asparagus.

3. Gather edges of parchment up over salmon and tie tightly with kitchen twine to form sealed pouch.

4. Place pouch directly on hot baking sheet in hot oven. Bake for 20 minutes.

5. Remove from oven and carefully transfer pouch to serving plate. Carefully open pouch to release steam.

6. Serve hot.

Snack Ideas

Sausage And Peppers

Prep Time: 5 minutes

Cook Time: 10 minutes

Servings: 4

INGREDIENTS

4 Italian sausage links (pork, chicken, etc.)

1 white onion

1 bell pepper

INSTRUCTIONS

1. Heat large skillet over medium heat. Add 1 tablespoon coconut oil.
2. Peel onion. Stem and seed pepper. Roughly chop onion and pepper. Slice sausage into 3/4 inch slices.
3. Add sausage to hot oiled skillet and sauté about 2 minutes. Then add onion and peppers. Sauté about 8 minutes, until sausage is cooked through and browned.
4. Serve hot.

Spicy Chicken Bites

Prep Time: 5 minutes

Cook Time: 10 minutes

Servings: 4

INGREDIENTS

8 oz boneless skinless chicken

1/2 cup almond meal

1 teaspoon flax meal

1 teaspoon paprika

1/2 teaspoon cayenne pepper

1/2 teaspoon red pepper flakes

1/2 teaspoon ground black pepper

1/2 teaspoon sea salt

1 egg

1 jalapeño pepper

2 garlic cloves

2 oz organic spicy brown mustard

Coconut oil (for cooking)

INSTRUCTIONS

1. Heat a medium skillet over medium high heat. Lightly coat pan with coconut oil.

2. Slice chicken into 1x1 inch strips. Arrange slices between 2 sheets of parchment and pound with kitchen mallet or rolling pin to flatten slightly. Place flattened pieces between two paper towels to absorb excess moisture.

3. In a shallow dish, blend almond meal, flax meal, dry spices and salt.

4. Add egg , jalapeño and peeled garlic to food processor or bullet blender. Process until fairly smooth. Pour into shallow dish.

5. Dip chicken pieces into jalapeño egg, then dredge in seasoned almond meal.

6. Carefully place coated chicken pieces into hot oil and fry about 2 minutes, until golden brown and cooked through. Turn with tongs half way through.

7. Drain cooked chicken on paper towel, then transfer to serving dish.

8. Serve hot with spicy mustard.

Simple Guacamole

Prep Time: 5 minutes

Cook Time: 5 minutes

Servings: 4

INGREDIENTS

2 avocados

1 shallot

1 small tomato

1 bunch cilantro

Half lime

2 teaspoons paprika

1/2 teaspoon ground cumin

1/2 teaspoon ground black pepper

1/2 teaspoon sea salt

INSTRUCTIONS

1. Peel and finely dice shallot. Dice tomato and cilantro. Add to small mixing bowl.
2. Slice avocados in half, pit, and scoop flesh into bowl. Add 1 teaspoon paprika, 1/2 teaspoon cumin, 1/2 teaspoon black pepper and 1/2 teaspoon salt.
3. Mash avocado and mix ingredients well with fork. Transfer to serving dish and squeeze on juice of half a lime. Sprinkle with remaining teaspoon of paprika.
4. Serve immediately. Or refrigerate 30 minutes, and serve chilled.

Green Deviled Eggs 'N Ham

Prep Time: 5 minutes

Cook Time: 10 minutes

Servings: 4

INGREDIENTS

8 eggs

1 avocado

1/2 teaspoon ground black pepper

1/2 teaspoon salt

2 oz natural ham

2 tablespoons fresh dill

INSTRUCTIONS

1. Bring medium pot of lightly salted water to boil. Gently add eggs to hot water with tongs and cook about 8 - 10 minutes.

2. Drain eggs in colander and cool in cold water.

3. Crack shells and peel eggs. Cut eggs in half lengthwise and scoop out yolks into small bowl. Arrange whites on platter with center hollows facing up.

4. Mash avocado, salt and pepper with egg yolks until smooth. Dice ham and dill, separately.

5. Scoop avocado blend into each egg white hollow and sprinkle with ham, then dill.

6. Refrigerate about 20 minutes. Serve chilled.

Pigs In A Blanket

Prep Time: 20 minutes

Cook Time: 15 minutes

Servings: 4

INGREDIENTS

1 package(26 count) nitrate-free/nitrite-free mini hot dogs

3 egg whites

1/4 cup almond flour

1/4 cup coconut flour

1 tablespoon cold coconut oil

1/2 teaspoon baking powder

Pinch garlic powder

Pinch sea salt

2 oz organic mustard

INSTRUCTIONS

1. In separate medium bowl, mix almond and coconut flours with baking powder. Cut-in cold coconut oil, then add pinch of garlic powder and salt. Mixture should be crumbly. Refrigerate 15 - 20 minutes.
2. Preheat oven to 400 degrees F. Line sheet pan with parchment or lightly coat with coconut oil.
3. Whisk egg whites in medium bowl until white and frothy, just before soft peaks develop.
4. Gently fold egg whites into refrigerated flour mixture until just combined.

5. Flatten 1 level teaspoon of dough into a rectangle in your fingers. Place one sausage in middle of dough wrap it around the sausage. Repeat with remaining sausage and dough.
6. Place wrapped sausages on prepared sheet pan and bake about 15 minutes, until dough is golden brown and links are heated through.
7. Serve hot with mustard.